Polycystic Kidney Disease Diet

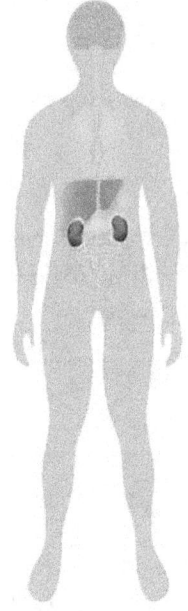

I0435649

Health Learning Series

M. Usman

Mendon Cottage Books

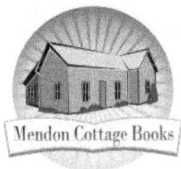

JD-Biz Publishing

Disclaimer

The information is this book is provided for informational purposes only. It is not intended to be used and medical advice or a substitute for proper medical treatment by a qualified health care provider. The information is believed to be accurate as presented based on research by the author.

The contents have not been evaluated by the U.S. Food and Drug Administration or any other Government or Health Organization and the contents in this book are not to be used to treat cure or prevent disease.

The author or publisher is not responsible for the use or safety of any diet, procedure or treatment mentioned in this book. The author or publisher is not responsible for errors or omissions that may exist.

Warning

The Book is for informational purposes only and before taking on any diet, treatment or medical procedure, it is recommended to consult with your primary health care provider.

Our books are available at
1. Amazon.com
2. Barnes and Noble
3. Itunes
4. Kobo
5. Smashwords
6. Google Play Books

Table of Contents

Polycystic Kidney Disease (PKD)

Chapter # 1: Overview

Kidneys are two extremely vital organs, each of the size of a person's fist located in the upper portion of a person's body. Precisely speaking, they lie in a person's abdomen, towards the back. The kidneys perform the complex task of filtering any type of waste product and/or toxics from the urine; secondarily they are also tasked with regulating the levels of certain hormones in the body.

Now that you know what kidneys are and what they do, you should be aware of cysts as well. Cysts are balloon-like, round structures that are filled with liquid. A moderate amount of these entities are considered normal in the kidney, but in PKD or Polycystic Kidney Disease, hundreds of cysts form in each kidney, giving birth to a problem that has become a serious issue in the 21st Century. Notice that cysts can form in other body organs as well, e.g. pancreas and liver, but are usually dormant.

Polycystic Kidney Disease

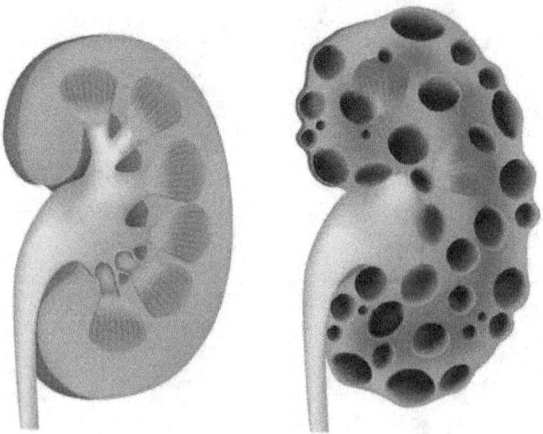

Polycystic kidney disease is a genetic disease that is characterized by the explosive growth of several cysts in a person's kidneys. A person may have PKD for several years and never notice, but when PKD causes kidneys to fail, the patient requires treatment in the form of either dialysis or kidney transplantation. Almost half the people, who have PKD, also have kidney failure; this condition is known as end-stage renal disease. PKD can also become the source of other problems by causing cysts in the liver, brain, heart, and blood vessels, which increases the complications to the existing disease.

In the United States alone, almost 600,000 people have Polycystic Kidney Disease, and it is categorized as the 4th leading cause of kidney failure. There are many forms to the disease but the 2 most common ones are:

i. Autosomal Dominant PKD:

This form of PKD is inherited from a family member. Symptoms to this type develop between the years of 30 and 40, but some also appear during childhood. About 90% of all cases are Autosomal Dominant.

ii. Autosomal Recessive PKD:

This is a rare yet inherited form of Polycystic Kidney Disease whose symptoms can appear as early as in a mother's womb.

More will be told about each type and ways to prevent it from occurring in later chapters. Primarily this book will focus on Autosomal Dominant Polycystic Disease as it is the most common occurrence of the disease.

Chapter # 2: Autosomal Dominant PKD

What is meant by Autosomal Dominant? The phrase means that if either parent has the disease, there is a 50 percent chance that the gene carrying the disease will be transferred to the child. In some rare cases, Autosomal Dominant PKD has been reported to occur spontaneously within patients; in this case neither of the parents carries the gene containing the disease.

Even though it is the most common type of inherited disorder in the kidneys, it certainly isn't the fastest one to strike; people with autosomal dominant PKD can live for quite a long time, e.g. several decades, without developing any symptom of the disease. It is for this very reason that autosomal dominant PKD is also called adult PKD. But still, rare cases have been spotted in which cysts appear early in childhood and start to show their signs quite earlier than predicted.

The cysts grow out of tiny filtering units within the kidneys known as nephrons. These cysts soon separate from the nephrons and continue to grow; along with these cysts the kidneys also become larger. In a fully developed autosomal domination PKD kidney, thousands of cysts are present. The kidney can weigh as much as 30 pounds and high blood pressure is common in these people.

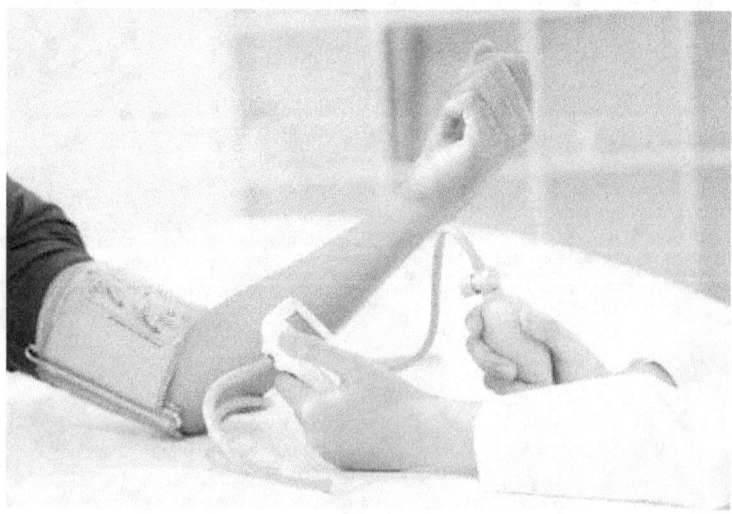

The most common and repeatedly occurring symptom of PKD is pain between the ribs and back, in the back, sides, and head. The pain may sometime be temporary but can also persist with intensity ranging from mild to high. Patients of autosomal dominant PKD may also experience the following signs:

- Urinary tract infections,

- Liver and pancreas cysts,

- Hematuria,

- Abnormal heart valves,

- Kidney stones,

- High blood pressure,

- Diverticulosis – bulges in the brain's blood vessel walls

- Aneurysms – bulge or bulges through the colon protruding outwards

Autosomal dominant PKD is diagnosed using advanced imaging techniques like CT scans and ultrasounds. The most common tool for diagnosing the kidney for PKD is ultrasound, but precise tools like CT scanners also exist which can tell more detail about the organ. The condition of one's kidney can vary greatly depending on his/her age therefore doctors have set specific criteria for classifying a patient as PKD. For example, a person has PKD if there are at least 2 cysts in each kidney when a person is 30 and his family medical history is also filled with the disease. However, in most cases of PKD, patients have no symptoms at all and their physical condition appears extremely normal; the disease thus goes unnoticed. Physical checkups, like urine and blood tests, may also not confirm the presence of this disease therefore PKD continues to go unnoticed for several decades. But once the cysts grow to about ½ an inch, diagnosis tools can reveal the identity of the disease. Ultrasound is the most commonly used imaging tool for the diagnosis due to its low safety concerns compared to other methods; it is also highly accurate as it can detect cysts inside a fetus!

Diagnosis may also be made using genetic testing to identify mutations in the Autosomal dominant PKD genes called PKD2 and PKD. Although this test is very useful in detecting the disease before large cysts develop, its usefulness is limited by the fact that detection does not tell about the severity of the disease or the time when it is going to cause the most damage. Still, a young adult who knows about the presence of genes within him can forestall the complete onset of PKD by following a healthy lifestyle.

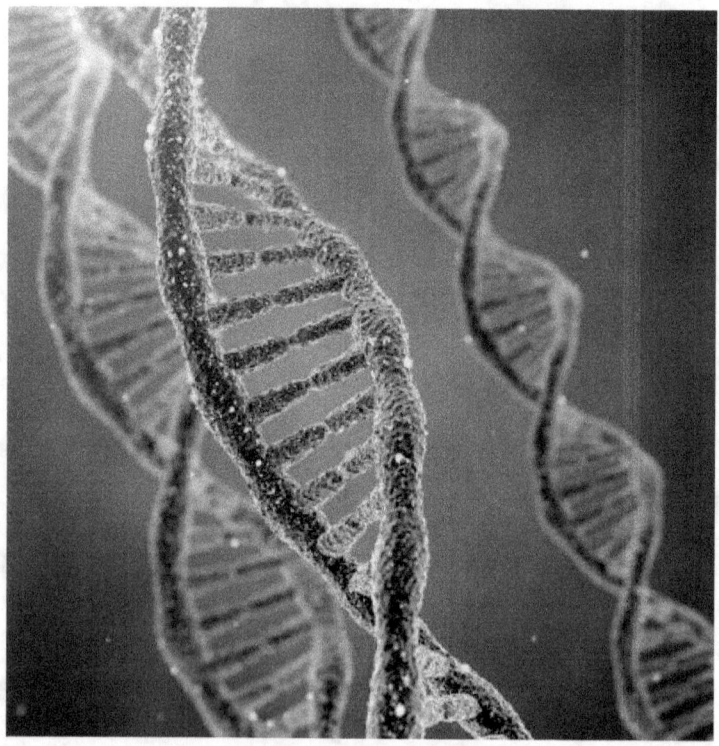

Chapter # 3: Autosomal Recessive PKD

Autosomal recessive PKD is the second most common type of PKD and is caused due to genetic mutation in the autosomal recessive PKD gene known as PKHDL. Furthermore, scientists believe more genes exist that support PKD, but until now only one has been found.

We all carry 2 instances of every gene; if both parents carry a copy of the abnormal gene and both pass this gene onto their child then the child has PKD. The chance of the child having autosomal recessive PKD gene is almost 25 %. Note that if only one parent has an abnormal gene, the baby can never have autosomal recessive PKD, but can only pass the gene onto his/her children.

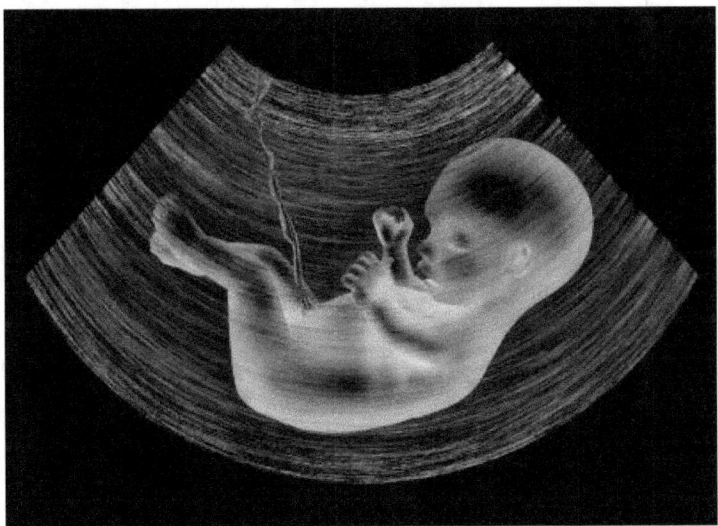

The signs of autosomal recessive PKD begin way before birth, in the mother's fetus. This is known as infantile PKD. Children that are born with this disease might not always develop failure of kidneys before they reach adulthood. The severity however varies; babies with the worst cast die within hours of their deliveries, due to respiratory difficulties. Just like the former case, some people with autosomal recessive variant do not develop signs of the disease until decades later. Liver scarring starts in sufferers of autosomal recessive PKD and keeps on getting worse with the passage of time.

Symptoms of autosomal recessive PKD are urinary tract infections, high blood pressure, and frequent urination. The disease also affects the spleen and the liver resulting in a lower number of blood cells, hemorrhoids, and varicose veins. Because the function of kidneys is vital during early stage of a child's growth, children with autosomal recessive PKD are smaller in size compared to average children.

Ultrasound imaging is used to reveal enlarged kidneys in a newly born child or in the fetus; some cysts are often missed so the liver is often checked for scarring damage as it is another sign of autosomal recessive PKD.

Autosomal recessive PKD is often treated with antibiotics and other drugs that control urinary tract infections and high blood pressure. In some cases growth hormones are also used for treatment. In cases of kidney failure, autosomal recessive PKD is treated via transplantation or dialysis whereas in extreme cases a combined liver + kidney transplant takes place.

PKD Diet

Chapter # 1: Intro

People with PKD, either type, have to make quite frequent visits to the doctor depending on the degree of damage caused by the cysts. There is currently no treatment or sure cure for the disease or any under development so the only current treatment is prevention. Prevention is aimed at controlling the signs and symptoms and complete outbreak of cysts in the kidney.

- By following a healthy diet pattern, performing regular exercises and keeping good weight.

- Monitoring and keeping blood pressure in check as high blood pressure causes the kidney function to reduce.

- Monitoring your cholesterol levels.

So far the first technique has proven the most effective as it equally treats high blood pressure and cholesterol levels as much as it treats PKD.

Chapter # 2: What is it?

The function of kidneys is to purify the body of waste products like acidic waste; what polycystic kidneys do is that they produce more acidic waste than the kidneys can actually process. Firstly, doctors will give these patients alkalizers when the function of kidneys has been greatly diminished. Medical research conducted by Tanners has also shown that when an alkaline diet was given to PKD models, the growth of cysts in kidneys was delayed. Alkalinity not only kept the polycystic kidneys from enlarging, but also extended the lives of the kidneys and allowed it to thrive for twice as long. Thus it is proven that a non-acidic diet is the way to go.

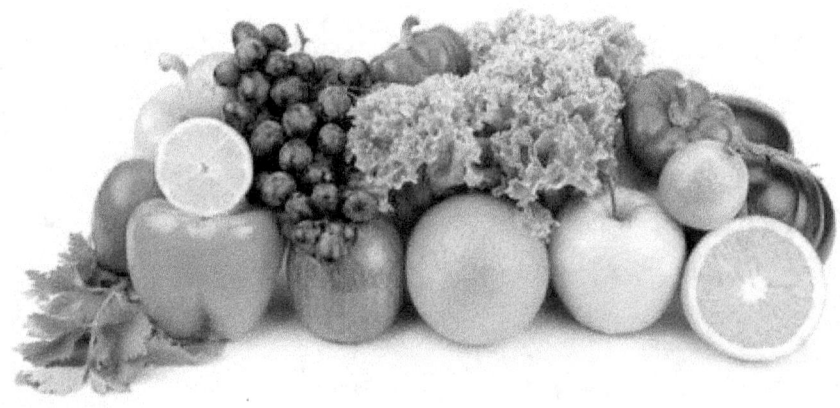

Although there is no fixed PKD Diet, there is hope that a diet directed towards cystic kidney health could decrease the patient's chances of organ failure. Basically, an alkaline diet is the key, therefore a low salt, neutral protein diet coupled with sufficient amount of water. Too much salt can raise blood pressure which can put extra pressure on the kidneys. Keep your daily aim to intake less than 5 grams of salt; this 5 grams represents the whole daily intake including, foods with hidden salts like ham, sausages and ready-to-cook meals. You can easily record the amount of salt contained within a food item by looking at the packet details. Salt may be listed as sodium in which case 1 g of sodium is equal to 2 g of salt. Also avoid "low salt" products as they contain potassium which is harmful to kidneys.

Most common examples of alkaline foods include fruits and vegetables so feel free to eat them as much as you can. Generally, the sweeter the vegetable or fruit, the more alkaline it is. Fruits and veggies are also a great source for replenishing one's vitamins and mineral supplies that can help regulate blood pressure. Aim for 5 portions of fruits and vegetables every day; try to increase the servings if possible.

Acidic foods include animal proteins which should be eaten in a controlled quantity. If one can eliminate these proteins then it is much better, but in order to obtain the essential fatty acids and amino acids, some protein must go in. If you can't completely adjust to plant based foods and must include something else, then limit yourself to lamb, broths, soft white cheese, egg yolk, and white fish, and keep the intake checked to less than three ounces each day with a frequency lower than two times a week. Another approach to consuming protein is that for every kilo of your body mass eat 1 grams protein from fish and from meat carrying low amounts of saturated fat. Furthermore, you may eat more protein if you are doing some hard labor.

Plant based proteins may be consumed if you are a vegetarian like spelt, sweet potatoes, carrot juice, corn, cabbage juice, chia seeds, beans, nuts, grains, legumes and seeds. Soak the nuts before cooking them as this will decrease their phytic acid content which will not only increase their alkalinity, but also enhance their digestibility.

Maintaining your fluid intake is also very important; drink at least 10 glasses of fluid each day, excluding alcohol! Polycystic kidneys are less efficient at retaining water so beware of this problem.

Alcohol won't damage your kidneys as it is the task of your liver to remove alcohol from the body, but it would definitely work against the factors keeping kidney failure at bay. Thus, the recommended limits for alcohol are:

i.   2 – 3 alcohol free days per week.

ii. 2 – 3 units a day for women.

iii. 3 – 4 units per day for men.

Too much alcohol is unhealthy for you because:

- These drinks contain a hefty amount of calories which can make it harder for you to keep extra weight off.

- Alcohol raises your blood pressure that increases the risk of kidney failure.

- It causes liver problems.

- It can interfere with some prescription medications.

- It increases the risk of cancers.

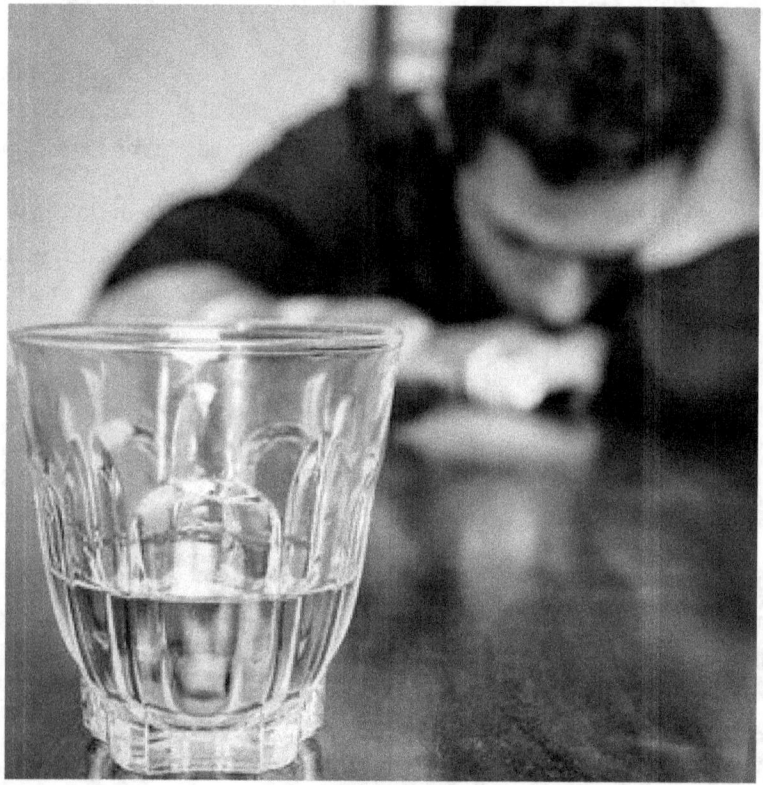

Smoking is injurious for anyone and not just a sufferer of Polycystic Kidney Disease. Smoking damages the kidney by shooting up the blood pressure that not only aids in kidney failure, but also increases the risk of strokes and heart failure.

It must be kept in mind that unlike alcohol, these substances are removed from the bloodstream via kidneys. Many have multiple effects on the body thus it is beneficial for the body to have the least amount of drugs in it as possible.

Along with following a healthy diet pattern, it would be very advantageous to exercise regularly as it will help you to control your blood pressure and weight, which will ultimately protect your kidneys. Aim for at least 30 minute of physical activity five times a week; so that you feel shortness of breath. Try to find an activity you enjoy so that you do not feel stressed out; try to avoid any contact sports like boxing, hockey, or rugby as it would increase the chances of a cyst bursting in your body!

Entrees

Chapter # 1: Black Bean Enchiladas

Ingredients for Black Beans:

- 1 cup black beans

- 2 minced garlic cloves

- ½ onion, chopped

- ½ carrot, diced

- Ground pepper

- Cilantro

- Himalayan salt

- ½ teaspoon cumin

Directions for Black Beans:

Soak the beans in water and keep rinsing them with running water every morning; fresh water should be used. On the third day, cook the beans alongside diced carrots and chopped onion; bring them to a boil and let them simmer for an hour.

Directions for Enchiladas:

Preheat an oven to 350 degrees Fahrenheit. Next, heat the tortillas until they are soft; take one at a time. Take a tortilla and add a spoonful of black beans, raw onions, some corn, slices of avocado, and a few chopped olives. Roll them into cylindrical shape and place all of them in an oven proof container. Carry the same steps with all the tortillas. Place any leftovers like onions, olives, and corn on top if desired. Cook the carrots and place them in a blender, pureeing them thinly. Season and place 2-3 tablespoons of carrot puree over them. Place the enchiladas in the preheated oven for about 15 minutes. When they are done, sprinkle cilantro over them and serve.

Ingredients for Cashew Cream:

- 1 cup soaked cashews

- 1 teaspoon oregano leaves

- 2 garlic cloves

- ¼ cup water

Directions for Cashew Cream:

Soak the cashews for at least 2 hours. Use either a high speed blender or a food processor to blend the cashews, oregano, and garlic along with water. Pour this cream over the enchiladas with cilantro and avocado slices.

Chapter # 2: Raw-Food Mac & Cheese

Ingredients for Noodles:

- 1 zucchini

Directions for Noodles:

Process the zucchini through a slicer to create long noodles. Toss onto them some salt and let them sit for 45 minutes while preparing the rest of the recipe.

Ingredients for Cheese Sauce:

- 2 tablespoon lemon juice

- 2 tablespoon water

- 1 ¾ cup cashews soaked for 1 – 2 hours

- 1 teaspoon Himalayan salt

- ½ clove garlic

- 1 teaspoon black pepper

- ¼ medium shallot

- A pinch of turmeric

Directions for Cheese Sauce:

Blend all of the ingredients, except the noodles, in a blender at high speed until they are completely smooth.

Ingredients for Mac & Cheese:

- Squash noodles, prepared above

- Cashew cheese sauce prepared above

- Chopped walnuts

- Himalayan salt

- Grinds of pepper mil

Directions for Mac & Cheese:

Toss the blended cashew sauce so that it lightly coats the noodles. Top it up with chopped walnuts and a few herbs; season & serve.

Chapter # 3: Beet Patties

Ingredients:

- 1 bay leaf

- ½ cup dried chickpeas soaked for 7 – 8 hours

- ½ cup quinoa

- 1 – 2 medium sized red beets

- 1 diced, medium sized onion

- 2 cloves garlic

- Himalayan salt

- 2 tablespoon lemon juice

- Zest of 1 lemon

- Juice of 1 lemon

- 1 egg

- ½ cup oats

Directions for Noodles:

Firstly, drain the chickpeas previously soaked and rinse them under the spigot. If you have an excess amount of time, soak the chickpeas once again and keep repeating the draining procedure for the next 3 days. Now place the chickpeas in a medium sized saucepan along with the bay leaf. Cover with at least 3 inches of water and bring it to a boil; reduce the heat and let it simmer until the beans turn tender. Next, add ½ teaspoon of the salt and continue cooking until the beans turn greatly tender but do not fall apart. This may take a variable amount of time, from 30 – 60 minutes depending on the quality of the beans. Add water as needed and after the beans are done, let them cool off, in their own water.

Place the quinoa in a fine mesh strainer; place this strainer in a bowl and fill this bowl with enough water so the quinoa is covered. Let the quinoa soak in the water for 5 – 10 minutes, giving it occasional swings so the bitter coating washes off. When the water turns beige-yellow in color, drain the quinoa and discard the water. Place the collected quinoa in a small sized saucepan and add a cup of fresh water and ¼ teaspoon salt. Bring this mixture to a boil, and immediately reduce the heat to low. Cover the pot and let the quinoa steam for 15 – 20 minutes or until it turns tender. Remove from the heat and let it sit for some time.

Next, peel the beets using a peeler and then grate them on well-sized holes. Wear an apron and cover anything you want to keep clean beforehand as the beets will spray when you grate them. Heat the oil in a sauté pan and as soon as it shimmers add onions and cook until they turn tender; this usually takes 5 – 10 minutes. Add the grated beets, garlic, and salt and once again give it a stir, covering the pan and letting the mixture cook for 5 – 10 minutes or until the beets turn tender. Remove the pan from heat and add two tablespoons of the lemon juice; stir up the pan and make sure nothing is stuck at the bottom. Next, divide the mixture into 6 portions; each of equal shape and size. Mold each portion into 1 thick round patty. Coat the bottom of a skillet with oil and turn on the heat. Carefully add the patties and cook until both sides are golden; each side would take 2 – 3 minutes to completely cook. Immediately reduce the heat if the burger turns brown too quickly.

Serve the burgers over buns alongside radish, sprouts, avocado, and mustard or with onion gravy.

Chapter # 4: Vegan Lasagna

Ingredients for Lasagna:

- ½ pounds fresh mushrooms, sliced

- 1 chopped onion

- 6 garlic cloves, chopped

- ½ cup parsley, chopped

- ¼ cup parsley, dried

- Pesto sauce

- 2 tablespoon water

- 2 teaspoon basil

- Almond cheese, grated

- Spelt lasagna

- ½ cup black olives, sliced

Ingredients for Filling:

- ¼ cup almonds

- 6 cups fresh spinach

- 1 teaspoon Himalayan salt

- ¼ cup almond milk

- 1 teaspoon basil chiffonade

- 1 ½ teaspoon marjoram

- ½ teaspoon minced garlic

- Ground pepper

Directions:

Preheat the oven to 375 degrees Fahrenheit. Start by sautéing the mushrooms, parsley and onion over medium heat in 2 tablespoons of water. Cover the container in between stirs to keep it from getting dry. Remove from heat after sautéing and add the sauce, basil, marjoram, and oregano. As the sauce starts to cool, add in the pressed or chopped garlic. Taste and add more garlic if desired. Put the ingredients for the filling in a food processor.

In a well-sized pan, boil the lasagna until it is greatly tender or just before they completely become al dente; this would take 8 – 9 minutes. Spread about half of the pesto or tomato sauce at the bottom of a 9x12 inches pan and place a single layer of noodles length wise over it, using two or three noodles; leave a little space in the middle. Spread half of the spinach filling on the noodles and add another layer of noodles. Top it up with sauce and add a third layer of noodles along with the sauce. Add olives to top it up.

Cover and bake the layers in the preheated oven for 30 minutes at 375 degrees. After 30 minutes, remove the lid and sprinkle with almond grated cheese and bake for 10 more minutes. Finally let it stand for 15 minutes and serve with salad or spelt bread.

Chapter # 5: Kabocha Squash Risotto

Ingredients for Noodles:

- 5 cups vegetable stock

- ¼ teaspoon saffron

- Olive oil spray

- Water with saffron

- 2 cups shitake, sliced thinly

- 4 stalks thyme leaves, fresh

- 1 teaspoon dried thyme

- ¼ teaspoon ground pepper

- ½ teaspoon Himalayan salt

- 1 cup brown rice

- 3 cups Kabocha squash

- ½ cup shelled pistachios

Directions for Noodles:

The skin of the squash is very tough and thus difficult to remove. Some people prefer the use of a rubber mallet to remove it while there is a much simpler way. Bring an 8 quart pot of water to a complete boil and add the squash. Let the squash boil uncovered for 3 minutes. Use tongs to flip the squash and boil for another 3 minutes. Drain and let it cool. Once cool enough, cut off both the top and the bottom and remove the skin using a paring knife. Cut the squash and scoop out all the seeds; cut the flesh into 1-inch pieces.

Place the broth with saffron in a medium-sized saucepan and bring it to a simmer. Reduce the heat so that the broth doesn't stop steaming. Spray a separate pan with olive oil and add shallots to it. Cook until they are fragrant; add thyme, mushrooms, salt, and pepper in it while cooking. Add the rice and vermouth and keep on stirring until it is absorbed. Add the remaining 3 cups of roasted squash and add in half a cup of saffron broth; keep adding half cups of stocks and continue to stir until the rice turns very creamy and consistent; all this would take 45 minutes. Once the risotto is soft and completely cooked, take off the heat and sprinkle cheese over it. Top it up with crushed pistachios and serve.

Others

Chapter # 1: Gluten-Free Sandwich Bread

Ingredients:

- 3 tablespoon Tupelo honey

- 3 cups gluten free flour blend

- 1 cup gluten-free sourdough starter

- 1 teaspoon Himalayan salt

- ½ cup warm almond milk

- 1 ¼ teaspoon guar gum

- 4 tablespoon olive oil

- 3 large eggs

Directions:

Place the honey, flour blend, salt, sourdough starter, and gum in a medium sized bowl and mix it well until all the contents of the bowl are smoothly combined. Use an electric mixer to drizzle the almond milk; the mixture will appear crumbly at first, but once the milk is added it will become of uniform texture. Add the olive oil to the mixture and beat it through a blender. Beat the eggs into the mixture, thoroughly beating them until they are all combined. Scrape the bottom as well as sides of the bowl and finally beat at medium to high speed for about 3 minutes; this will make the batter very smooth yet thick.

Next, cover the bowl with a plastic bag and let the batter thicken and rise for an hour. Scrape the bottom and sides of bowl while gently deflating the whole batter. Line a pan with parchment paper and scoop the dough into it. Press the dough to level it using a spatula or wet fingers. Cover this pan with a plastic bag and set it aside in a warm place until the bread crowns the rim of the pan. Let it rise for 60 minutes and towards the end of this time preheat an oven to 350 degrees Fahrenheit. Place the pan and bake the bread for 40 minutes or until it turns golden brown in color. After the designated time, remove it from the oven, place on a rack, and let it cool.

Chapter # 2: Apple Pie Pockets

Ingredients for crust:

- 2 ½ cup spelt flour

- 10 tablespoon coconut oil

- ½ teaspoon Himalayan salt

- ¼ cup ice-cold water

- ¼ cup additional water

Directions for crust:

Add the first four ingredients into a blender jar and secure with a lid. Pulse the ingredients 8 – 10 times; add ¼ cup water, securing the lid once again. Pulse 4 times, add the remaining water, and pulse again 4 times. Keep pulsing until dough is formed, and make sure that you don't over blend it. Remove the dough and divide it into two balls. Pat it into a smooth disc and wrap the dough in plastic, refrigerating for 2 hours before rolling it out. Roll out the dough after 2 hours and cut it into triangles, 17 – 20 if possible.

Ingredients for Pie filling:

- ½ cup "Just-like-brown-sugar"

- 1 tablespoon coconut oil

- 2 apples, sliced

- 1 teaspoon cinnamon, ground

- Some lemon juice to squeeze over the apples

Directions for Pie filling:

Add half of the apple into the jar and close the lid. Pulse 10 times and set it aside. Add the brown sugar, coconut oil, and cinnamon to a medium sized saucepan and heat it on a medium intensity stove until it melts; stir it frequently. Once the oil has melted, add the apples to the sauce pan and bring it to a boil. Turn down the heat and let the apples simmer for about five minutes. Next, put 1 ½ tablespoons of filling on 1 half of the triangle and fold the other half. Use a fork to press both the crusts and place these pockets on parchment paper that lines a cookie sheet. Bake in a preheated oven at 400 degrees Fahrenheit. Bake the pockets for 20 minutes or until they turn golden brown in color.

Chapter # 3: Lentil Sprouts Soup

Ingredients:

- 1 small onion, chopped

- ½ cup lentil sprouts

- 3 cloves garlic

- 1 carrot, chopped into cubic shape

- Bay leaf

- 3 tablespoon parsley, fresh

- Thyme

- 1 teaspoon cumin seeds, roasted

- ½ teaspoon mustard seeds, roasted

- 6 cups water

- Fresh turmeric, sliced

- Cinnamon stick

Directions:

Take out a stainless steel pressure cooker and sauté the garlic and onion in it for 2 minutes; add the bay leaf, thyme, carrot, mustard seeds, cumin seeds, cinnamon, and turmeric and keep sautéing until everything becomes fragrant. Next, add water to the pressure cooker and set it. Once the steam begins to come out, time it for 10 minutes. After 10 minutes, shut it down and allow it to cool on a natural pace, removing the lock. Taste the soup and season it if you want. If you're cooking on a stove top, then cook for 20 – 30 minutes. Part of the soup may be added to a blender if you consider it too thick; the blended soup may serve as a base for the rest of the soup. Once cooked, remove the turmeric and cinnamon stick; taste for seasoning. In order to bring the flavors together, squeeze fresh lemon juice over it. The soup may be served on its own or with brown rice or wild rice; it may also be eaten with bread if you want.

Conclusion

Some research centers have successfully carried out many studies and have identified the whole process that triggers the formation of cysts. Medical breakthroughs in the field of genetics are also proving fruitful and many scientists are working on a preemptive cure on PKD, while the child is still in the womb. But until these treatments get full confirmation from the medical world and federal institutions the only way to prevent a full blown PKD disease is by diet. As cysts are helped by an unhealthy life style and an unbalanced diet, the PKD can get worse over time. Thus, a low acidic diet should be followed which will keep the growth of cysts in check. Furthermore it would also alleviate symptoms that take extra pressure off kidneys like high blood pressure and cholesterol. The whole science behind the diet and the means to implement it has been given in the book. It's up to you to follow it and make a change in your life, for good.

Best of luck!

References

http://nl.123rf.com/photo_33572060_.html?term=Polycystic%20Kidney%20Disease

http://nl.123rf.com/photo_12176797_polycysteuze-nierziekte.html?term=Polycystic%20Kidney%20Disease

http://nl.123rf.com/photo_15398796_dubbele-dna-helix-moleculen-en-chromosomen.html?term=genes

http://nl.123rf.com/photo_20014989_zonsondergang-in-de-zomer-veld.html?term=ultrasound

http://www.fotolia.com/id/51912489

http://www.fotolia.com/id/45901427

http://www.fotolia.com/id/47136007

Author Bio

Muhammad Usman is a distinguished medical graduate of Allama Iqbal medical college (AIMC). He is a professional writer who has been in the field for more than 4 years. During this time he has produced 10,000+ articles, blogs, and eBooks on various niches related to diseases, health, fitness, nutrition, and well-being. He is a regular contributor to several journals related to medicine and surgery. He is the editor of several journals and newspapers.

Check out some of the other JD-Biz Publishing books

Gardening Series on Amazon

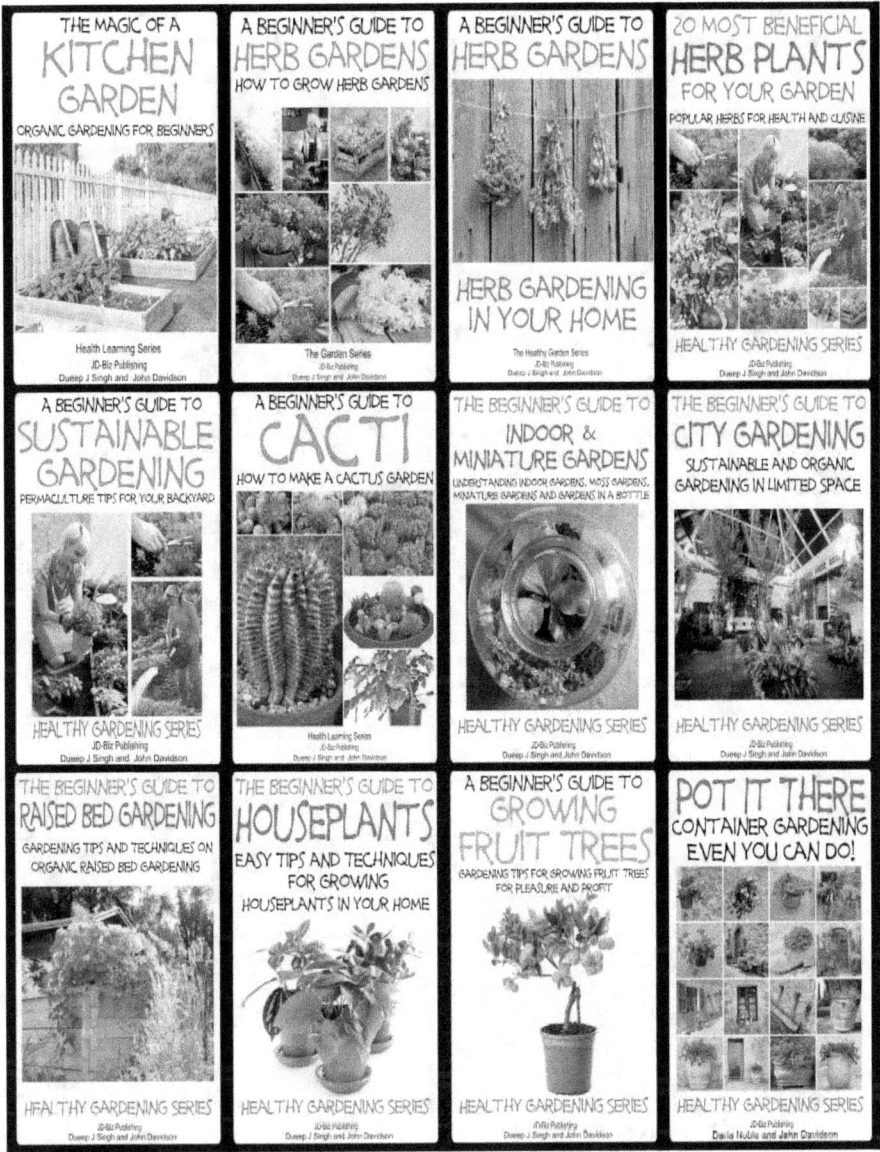

Health Learning Series

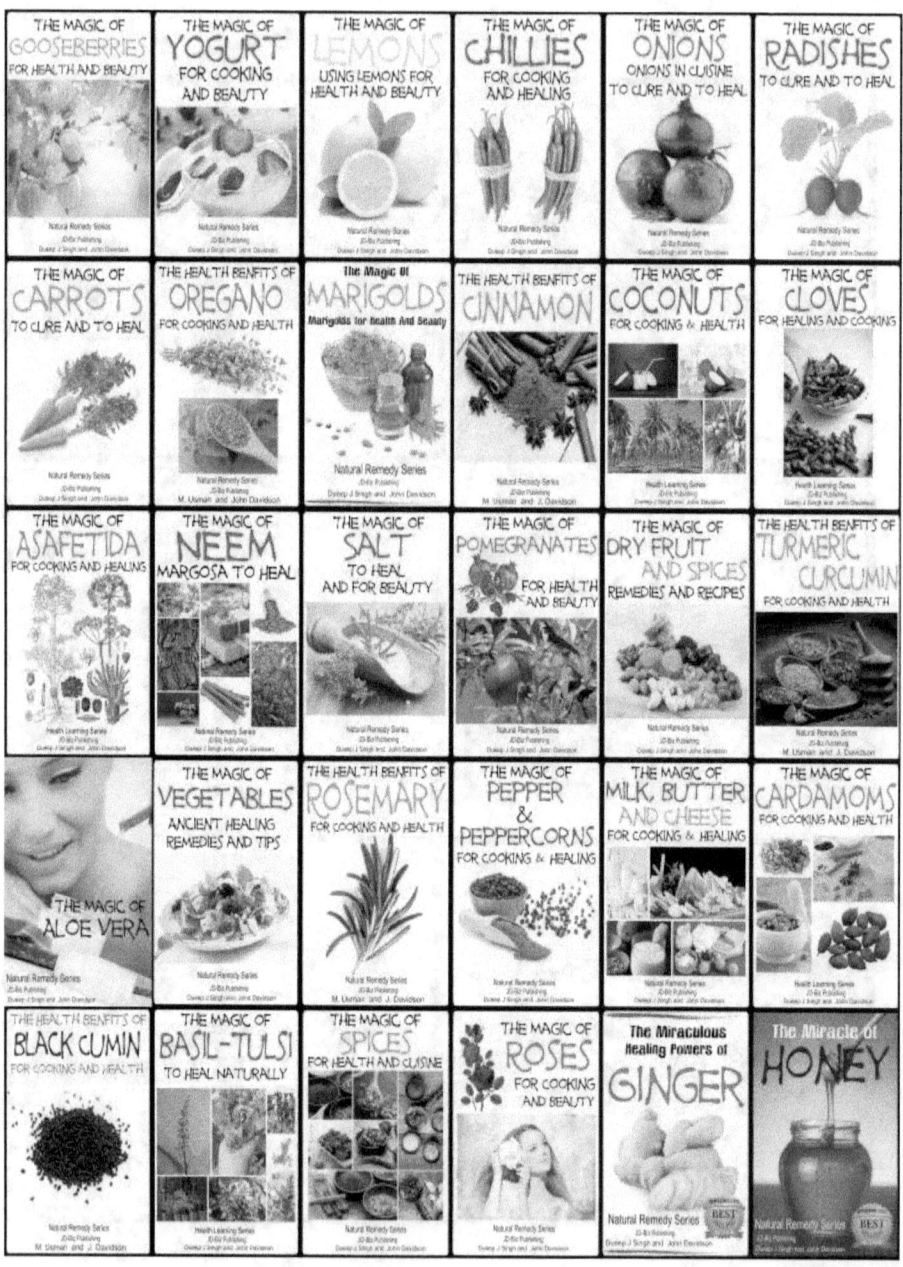

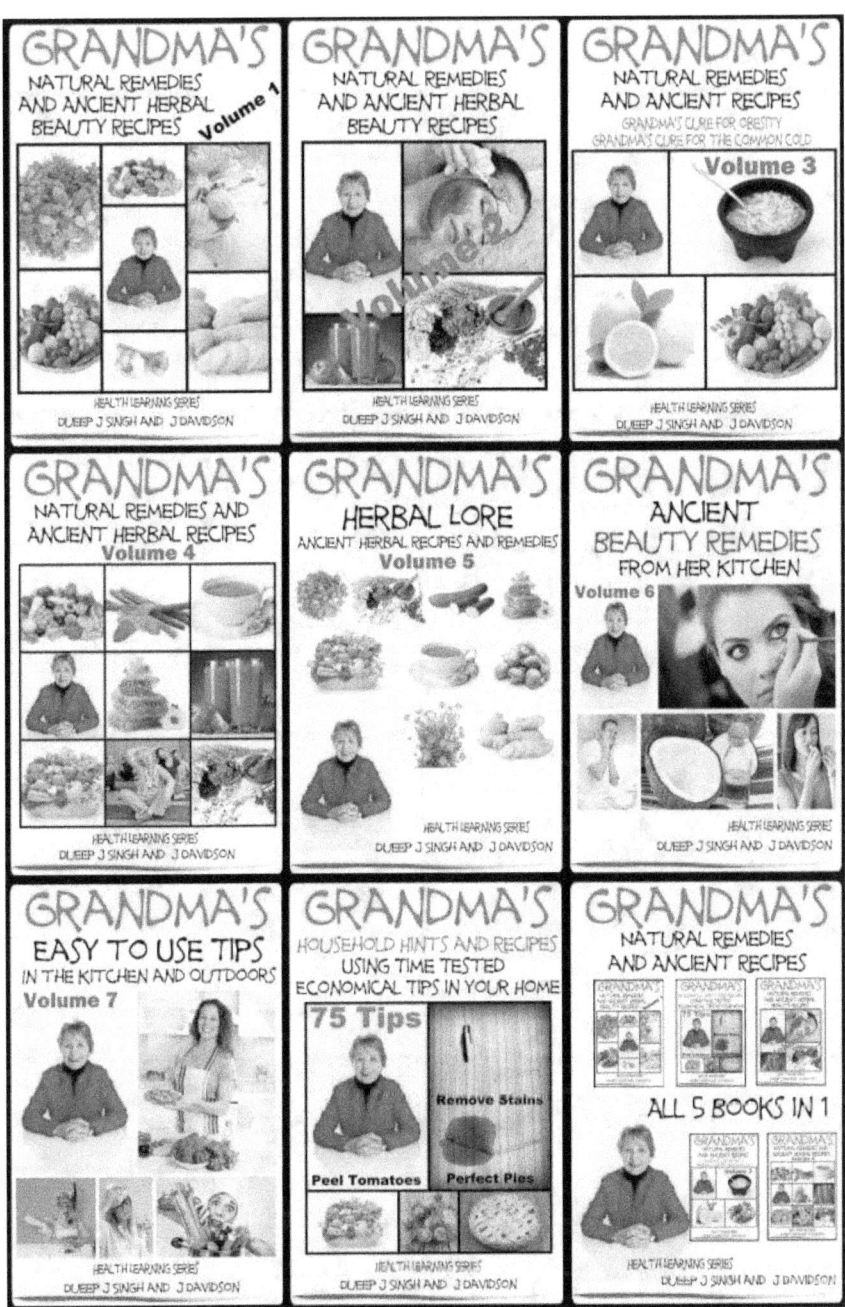

Country Life Books

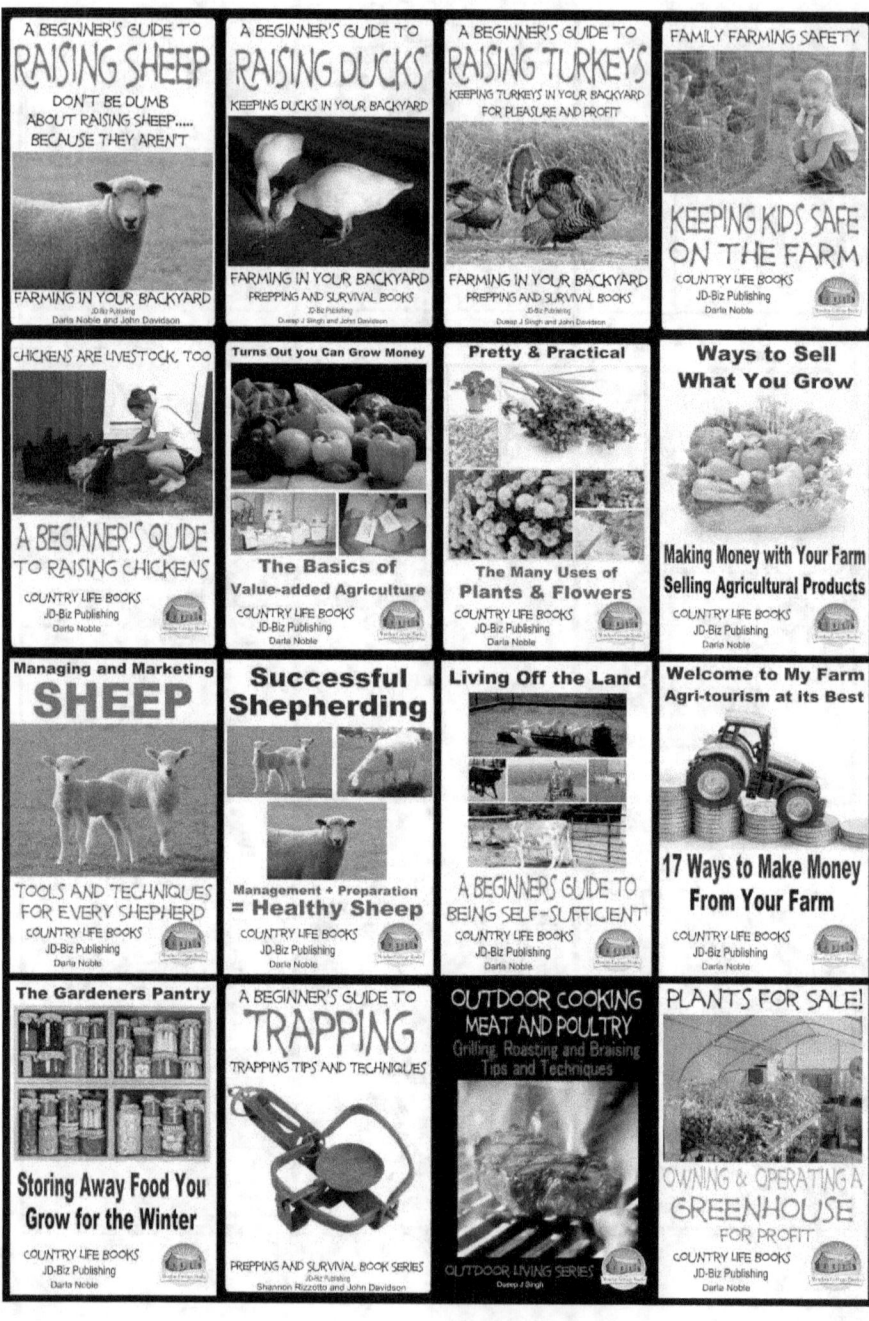

Health Learning Series

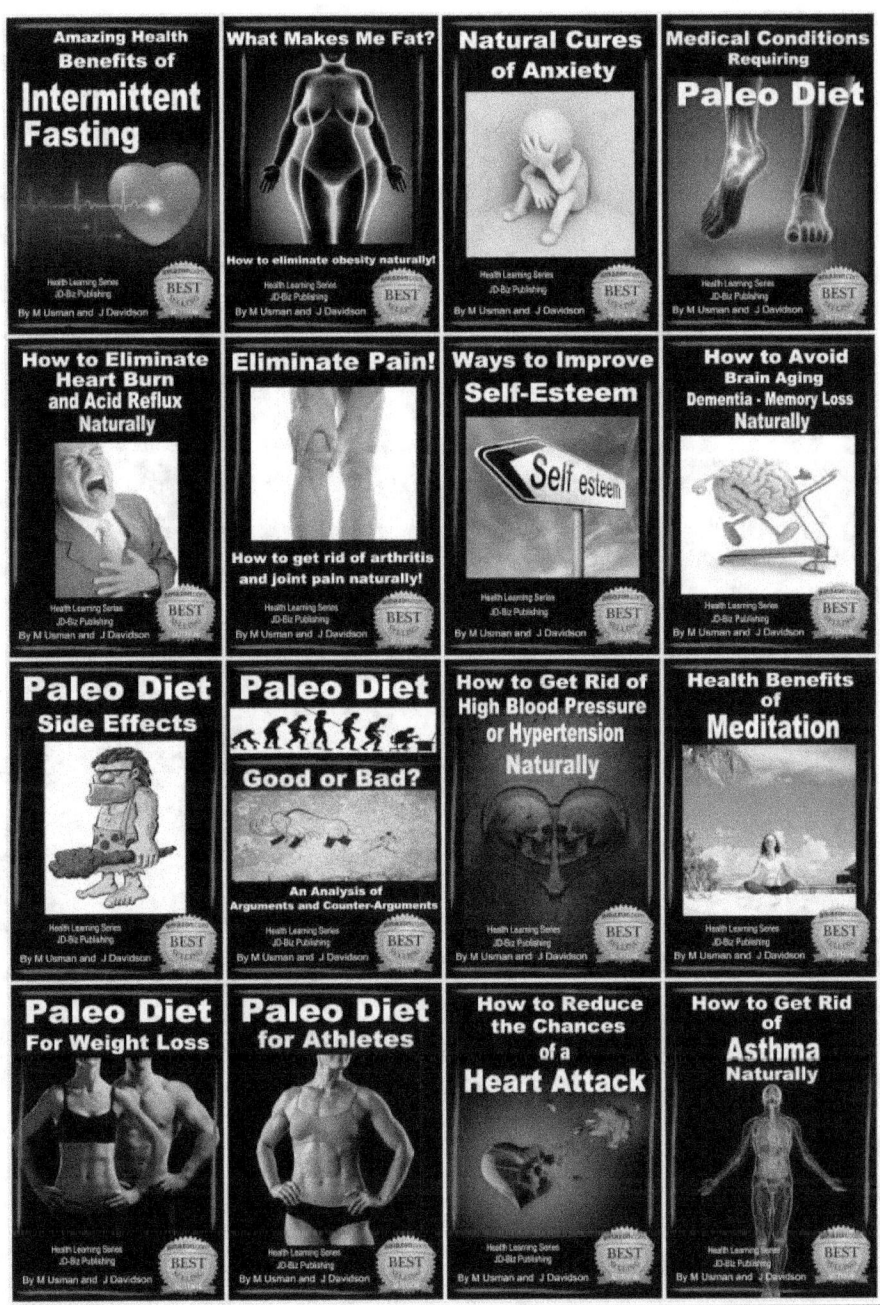

Amazing Animal Book Series

Learn To Draw Series

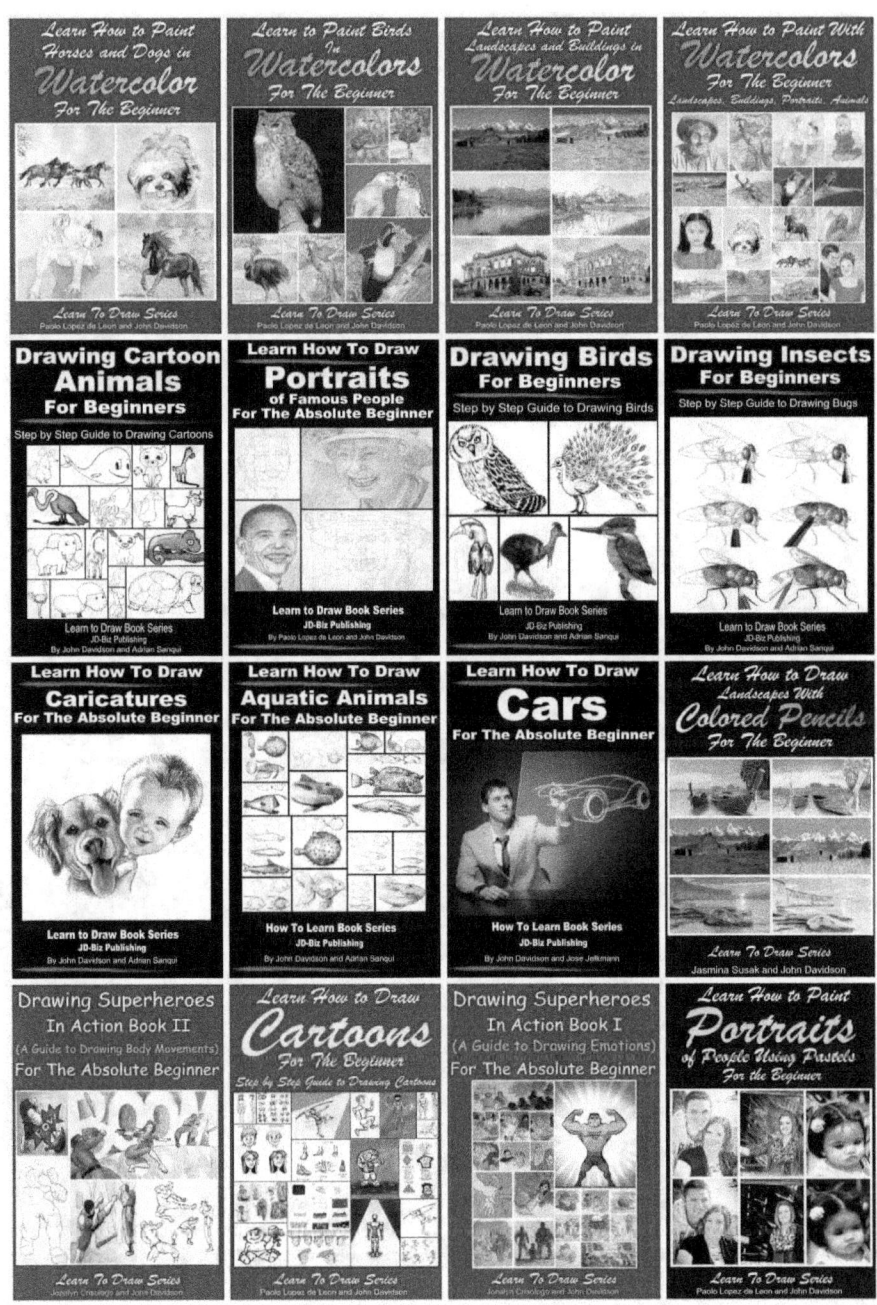

How to Build and Plan Books

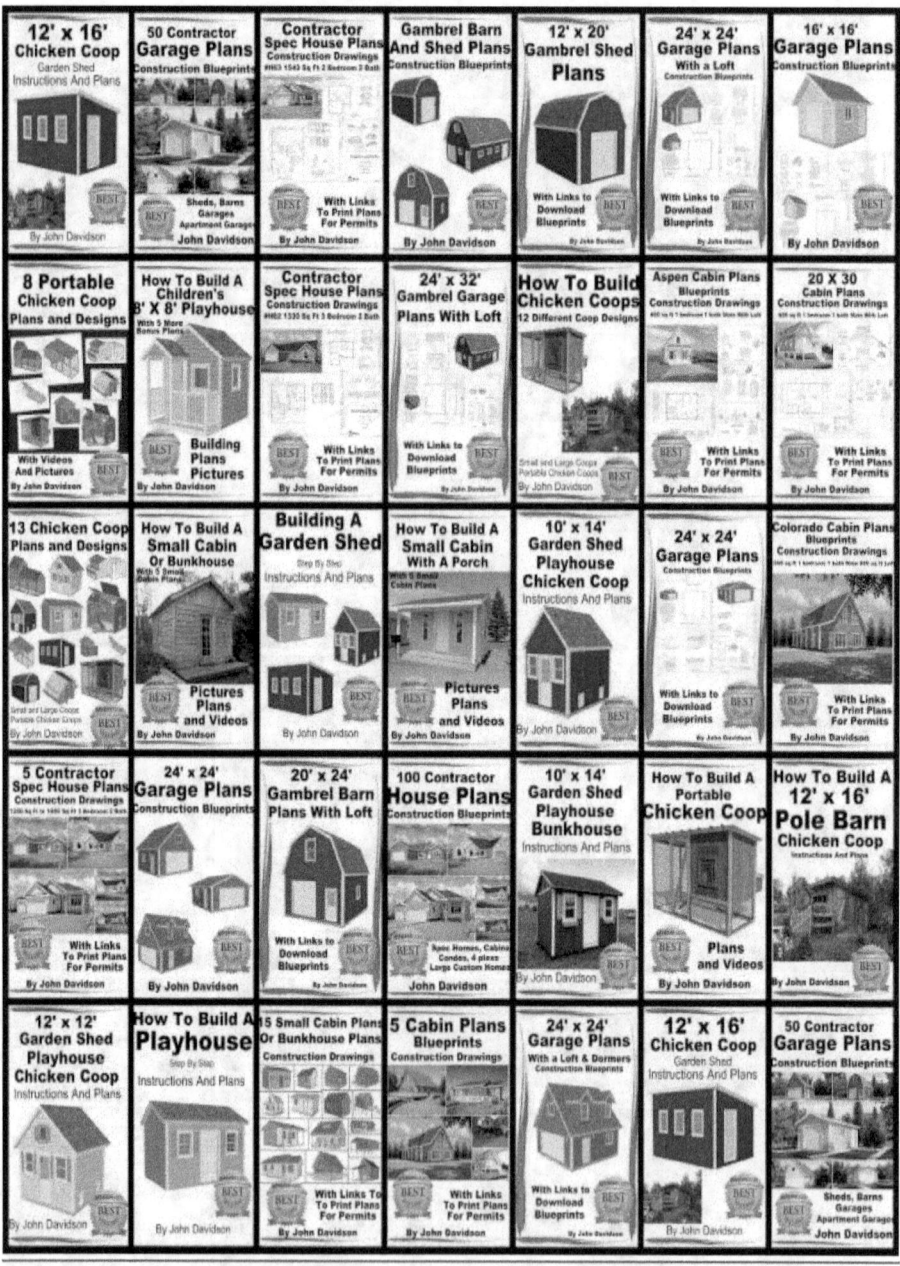

Entrepreneur Book Series

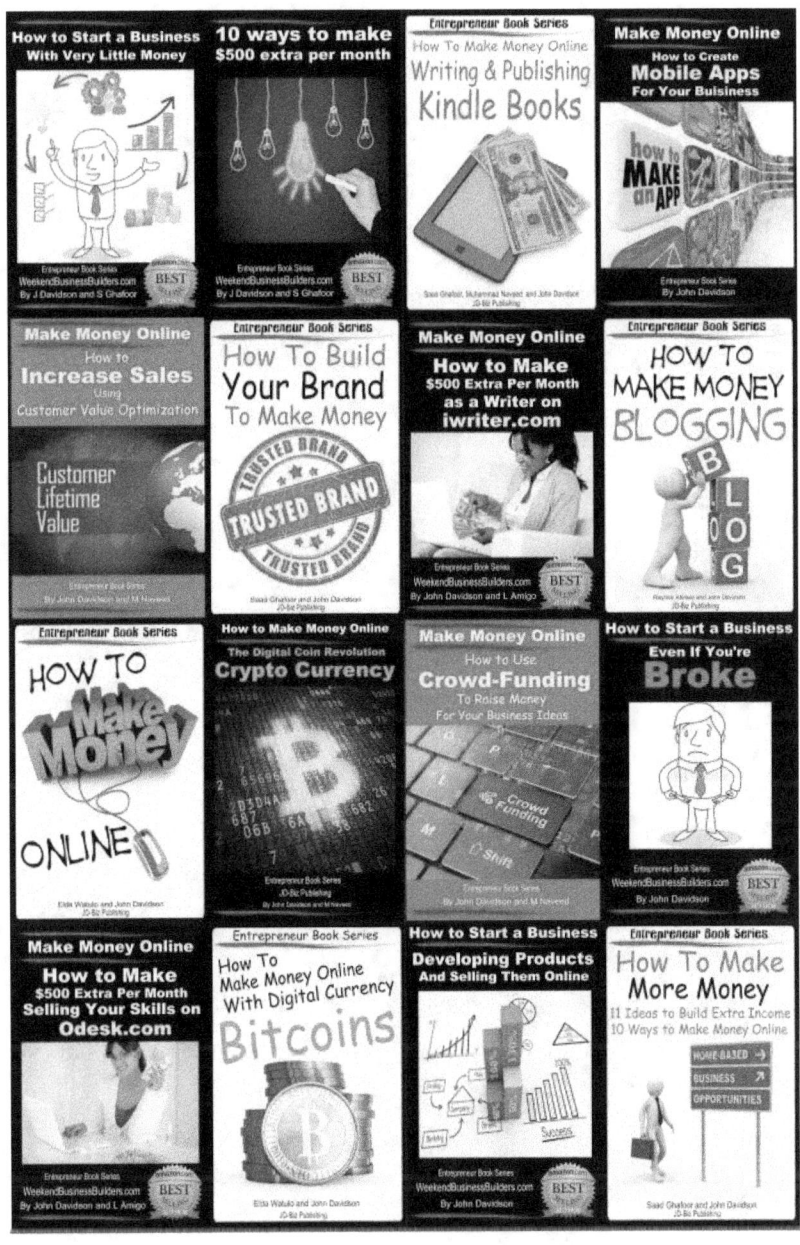

Our books are available at

1. Amazon.com

2. Barnes and Noble

3. Itunes

4. Kobo

5. Smashwords

6. Google Play Books

Publisher

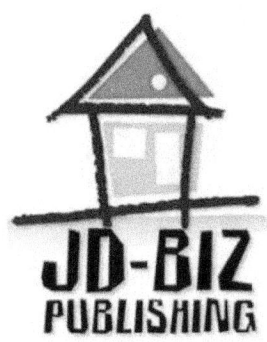

JD-Biz Corp

P O Box 374

Mendon, Utah 84325

http://www.jd-biz.com/

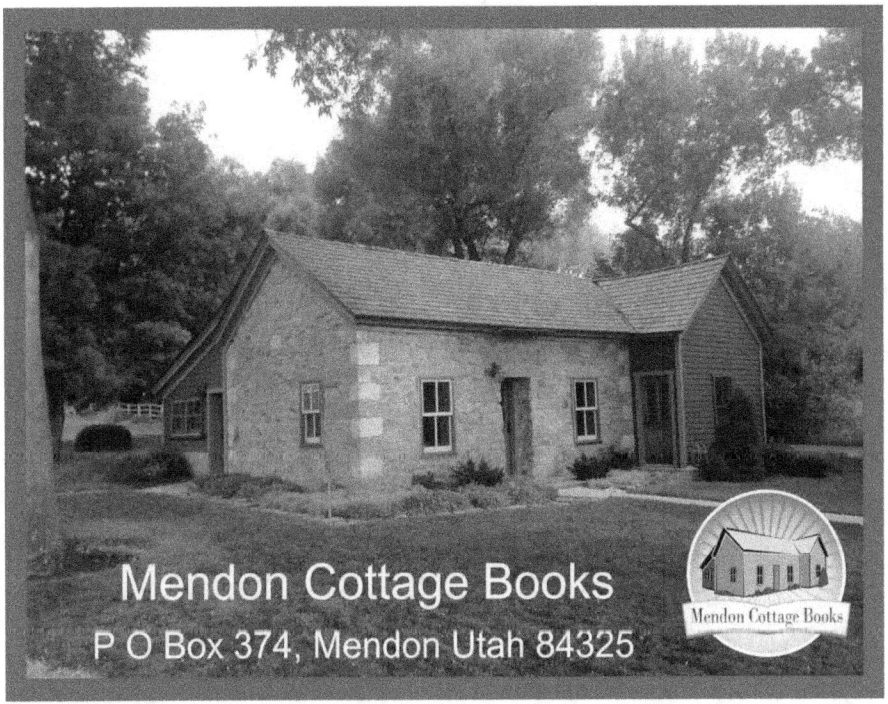

Mendon Cottage Books

P O Box 374, Mendon Utah 84325